the art
of
pole dancing

A Spin-by-Spin Guide

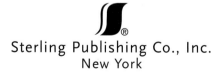

Sterling Publishing Co., Inc.
New York

Library of Congress Cataloging-in-Publication Data Available

10 9 8 7 6 5 4 3 2 1

Published by Sterling Publishing Co., Inc.
387 Park Avenue South, New York, NY 10016
© 2006 by Peekaboo Pole Dancing Ltd.
Distributed in Canada by Sterling Publishing
c/o Canadian Manda Group, 165 Dufferin Street
Toronto, Ontario, Canada M6K 3H6
Distributed in the United Kingdom by GMC Distribution Services
Castle Place, 166 High Street, Lewes, East Sussex, England BN7 1XU
Distributed in Australia by Capricorn Link (Australia) Pty. Ltd.
P.O. Box 704, Windsor, NSW 2756, Australia

Manufactured in the United States of America

Sterling ISBN-13: 978-1-4027-4238-5
         ISBN-10: 1-4027-4238-X

For information about custom editions, special sales, premium and
corporate purchases, please contact Sterling Special Sales
Department at 800-805-5489 or specialsales@sterlingpub.com.

Contents

the ART OF POLE DANCING

A Spin-by-Spin Guide

You've got it, so flaunt it

Welcome to Peekaboo Pole Dancing, the new form of pole dancing that's all about having sexy fun and flaunting everything you've got!

Pole dancing is hot right now—all the celebrities are doing it, people are doing it at parties, and classes are springing up everywhere. . . . But now it's your turn!

Becoming a Peekaboo Pole Dancer lets you show off your sexy side and have some uninhibited fun.

It's a great way to have fun with the girls, seduce the boys, or even give yourself a fun workout!

We believe there's a Peekaboo Pole Dancer in each of us. This book is going to help you find her!

WHAT IS PEEKABOO POLE DANCING?

Peekaboo Pole Dancing is a fun form of pole dancing that combines seductive poses with beginning moves, spins, and lifts. It can be used for both fun and fitness, and, like all dance forms, offers great freedom of expression. Peekaboo Pole Dancing has also been known to improve coordination and encourage improved self-confidence.

WHO PEEKABOO POLE DANCES?

Anyone! Women of all ages, shapes, and sizes can pole dance. Every woman has something worth flaunting, whether it's big breasts, skinny legs, a big booty, or even long hair. If there's music, you can use it. It's time to flaunt, flaunt, flaunt!

WHY PEEKABOO POLE DANCE?

Peekaboo Pole Dancing is becoming popular for three main reasons:

FLAUNTY FUN: Peekaboo Pole Dancing is a great way to lose your inhibitions, flaunt what you've got, and feel good about yourself. As well as learning a new skill, you'll experience a complete sense of freedom as you express your sexuality in a positive way. You'll also get the added benefit of feeling a little bit naughty, fun, and sexy all night long. These days you can pole dance at home, at bachelorette nights, at specialist classes, or even at your friends' parties! It's the ideal way to have a giggle, let your hair down, and put a little swing into the night.

SEXY FUN: If you have your own pole at home (or a prop that can be used as a pole), Peekaboo is a great way to heat things up in the bedroom. You'll be amazed how much your self-esteem and confidence grow as you begin to learn the moves and put together your own sexy routines. Take on your chosen Peekaboo persona (more on this later) and blow your partner's mind. Choose music and an outfit that complete the fantasy, and hold on tight! Prepare to get raunchy!

FITNESS: Wiggling and jiggling has never been so much fun. A good Peekaboo Pole Dancing session is equivalent to a fun workout. It's especially good for exercising all those sexy muscles that don't usually see the light of day, and it can be as easygoing or as strenuous as you want it to be. When the music starts pumping, so will your adrenaline!

So grab a pole, get hold of the nearest doorframe (or an obliging tall, skinny guy), and get to know a new and sexier you.

Peek-a-you!

Peekaboo Pole Dancing is all about you. About you having fun. About you feeling sexy. And about you showing off your hot body. It's time to free your inner Peekaboo Pole Dancer, lose all inhibitions, and go for it. Since it's all about you, it's important that you're in the right frame of mind before you start. Don't worry if you feel nervous or shy; everybody does at first. But once you get going, you'll find it a very liberating experience. As you learn the Peekaboo Pole Dance moves, your confidence will grow, and you'll enjoy it even more. After a while the moves will become second nature and won't seem so awkward! Remember, the key is to not take it too seriously, let your hair down, and have a giggle!

Which Peekaboo girl are you?

There are five different Peekaboo party-girl personas to help you get into the groove. Each girl has her own individual way of flaunting it and her own set of personal dance moves. You can dance as the girl who's most like you or have fun dancing as one of the others. It's entirely up to you!

GIRLY GIRL PINK

Transform yourself into Girly Girl Pink for the night and you're in for some good, clean, girly girl fun. She is the girliest and fluffiest of all the girls, and the one that likes to keep things cheeky . . . very cheeky.

Look: Girly Girl Pink likes to look girly. Keep makeup fresh, simple, and minimal—perhaps a light blusher and fake lashes to set hearts aflutter. Pigtails or ponytails are good.

Outfit: Pink T-shirts, skirts, nightshirts, teddies, and dresses are ideal. The pinker and cuter the better!

Music: Favorite Girly Girl Pink songs include "Barbie Girl" by Aqua, "The Look of Love" by Dusty Springfield, "Just My Imagination" by the Temptations, and "Love to Love You Baby" by Donna Summer.

Dancing: Dance moves should all be executed with a cheeky smile and a wink. Lots of teasing, shimmying, and especially wiggling are a particular pink preference!

Girly Girl Pink's pole dancing will have everyone tickled pink!

BABELICIOUS GIRL BLUE

Transform yourself into Babelicious Girl Blue for the night and enjoy the feeling of all eyes upon you. She is the Peekaboo girl who's all about looks. Her motto is "Look at me, look at me, look at me!" She loves to look her best at all times and loves the attention it brings even more.

Look: Babelicious Girl Blue likes to look good. She prefers to make the most of her features and brings them to life with lots of eye shadow (baby blue) and full-on lipsticks. Lip gloss is good for Peek-a-Pouting, and hair should be worn loose and free.

Outfit: Go for baby dolls, balcony bras, cutie-pie sets, halter tops, off-the-shoulder tops, and skirts that show plenty of thigh. Choose underwear that shows off your hot curves to the max and makes you feel like a million dollars. Outfits with flaunty, flirtatious frills are also particularly good.

Music: Babelicious Girl Blue loves songs she can pose and pout to. Her particular favorites include "Vogue" by Madonna, "Look at Me" by Geri Halliwell, "Hot Stuff" by Donna Summer, and "Word Up" by Cameo.

Dancing: Dance moves should be executed slowly and sensually, with a sexy pose and pout at the end of each. Be graceful and move at your own pace; the beautiful people rush for no one. Let your confidence flow with every sexy strut, turn, and twirl. Soak up the limelight and enjoying being center stage!

As Babelicious Girl Blue, you are the sexy superstar—strike a pose and dance like it!

PARTY GIRL PURPLE

Transform yourself into Party Girl Purple for the night and become the life and soul of the party. Party Girl Purple really likes to let her hair down and inject a little naughty fun into the proceedings. She gets the party started and keeps it started. Become Party Girl Purple and you'll get to enjoy the fun side of pole dancing. Don't take it too seriously, and have a giggle.

Look: Party Girl Purple likes to keep things sparkly! Glitter balm and party lashes are excellent Party Girl Purple accessories. Hair can be given the party treatment with a little added wave or curl.

Outfit: Party Girl Purple likes to dress up for a party! Party frocks, sparkly tops, and shimmering skirts are all fun. Anything with diamante is especially good at catching the party lights and making you look the party part!

Music: Party Girl Purple likes tunes that get people off their seats and on to the dance floor. Crowd pleasers and teasers are her specialty. Party favorites include "Get the Party Started" by Pink, "Spinning Around" by Kylie Minogue, "Rock Your Body" by Justin Timberlake, and "Play that Funky Music" by Wild Cherry.

Dancing: Use the pole as a very tall and shiny party accessory. Dance in a fun way, with energy and enthusiasm. Invite others to join in and perhaps give the shy ones a little extra encouragement. Enjoy the little spins and twists as you dance, and try to go with the flow. A few party drinks may help get you in the mood.

Dance as Party Girl Purple and soon the entire party will be getting into the swing.

GO-GO GIRL GREEN

Transform yourself into Go-Go Girl Green and let the music take control. She is the all-singing, all-dancing Peekaboo girl who likes nothing better than shaking her booty to the beat. Spin and high kick your way through track after track after track like a pole-dancing queen who's just got to be seen!

Look: Fitness is the vibe from Go-Go Girl Green. You'll be working up a sweat, so no need for any heavy makeup. Keep it fresh and simple and perhaps wear your hair tied back.

Outfit: Go-Go Girl Green likes to dance in whatever feels most comfortable. Mini skirts, hot pants, cropped T-shirts, leggings, and anything in figure-hugging Lycra is good. Comfortable footwear (no stilettos) is also recommended, as Go-Go Girl Green's routines can get a little frantic as she tries to keep up with the music.

Music: Go-Go Girl Green prefers funky, flaunty, booty-shaking beats. Go-Go Girl Green's favorite tracks are the ones that make you want to get out of your seat, grab a pole, and just dance. Let go of your inhibitions and let the music completely take over. Go-Go Girl Green's favorites include "Do a Little Dance" by KC and the Sunshine Band, "Bootylicious" by Destiny's Child, "Hung Up" by Madonna, "Dancing Queen," by ABBA, and "Jungle Boogie" by Kool & the Gang.

Dancing: Let yourself go and completely lose yourself in the music. Spin and shake to the beat, improvising your dance moves and routine where possible. Don't be afraid to improvise; there's no telling where the music is going to take you.

Become Go-Go Girl Green and Go-Go Get 'em!

BAD GIRL BLACK

Transform yourself into Bad Girl Black and become the baddest of all the bad girls. Bad Girl Black likes to misbehave and push things to the sexy limit. She's a sexy minx in the bedroom and specializes in devilishly dirty dancing.

Look: Bad Girl Black likes taking the bad-girl look to the extreme. Try wearing black eye shadow and black eyeliner coupled with dark-toned glossy lipsticks. If you can find one, a black bobbed wig can be an excellent addition.

Outfit: Black, black, and more black. Bad Girl Black likes wearing anything that's hot, sexy, and black. Black lingerie, slips, teddies, sexy dresses, stockings, stilettos, kinky boots, and G-strings are all ideal. PVC and rubber are also big favorites.

Music: Bad Girl Black music is music with attitude. It should be sexy and confident and allow the dancer to be firmly in charge. Bad Girl Black's favorites include "Dirty" by Christina Aguilera, "Tainted Love" by Marilyn Manson, "Bad" by Michael Jackson, and "Dirty Girl" by Beyonce.

Dancing: Dance slowly and sensually with a mischievous glint in your eyes. Maintain eye contact at all times, taking care to flaunt your sexiness to the max. Tease and toy with your audience and let them know who's in charge. If you're feeling really naughty, why not incorporate a striptease into your routine and lose an item of clothing or two! Feel free to set a bad example!

Become Bad Girl Black, grab your pole, and get ready to misbehave!

Peek-a-pointers

Before you get started, here are some Peek-a-Pointers to point you in the right direction.

Peek-a-Practice. Practice makes sexy! The more time you spend practicing, the more confident and comfortable you'll become around the pole. Confidence is everything!

Peek-a-Practice in front of a mirror to see how your moves look, and build up confidence.

Peek-a-Practice with your friends for extra-flaunty fun and encouragement.

To begin with, choose music you know well. This helps with confidence and makes planning your routine easier.

Look good and you'll feel good. Wear something that makes you feel sexy, and try to keep it practical. Hot pants, short skirts, and dresses that expose your bare legs and arms are ideal for feeling your way around the pole. Avoid outfits that are too tight or restrictive.

Go barefoot or wear running shoes until you feel confident enough for stilettos.

Perform moves that accentuate your favorite body parts. If you've got a big booty, then use it! Make the most of your legs, hair, hips, and anything else you want to flaunt!

Don't focus entirely on the dance pole. Try to see the pole and the area around it as your personal sexy play zone. Use the floor for sexy struts and flaunty floor moves.

Exaggerate and emphasize the sensual way you move your body. Shake, sway, shimmy, and wiggle things just that extra little bit for a sexier effect.

If you're dancing to seduce, try to maintain eye contact with your audience as much as possible.

Play with your audience. Tease them and toy with them. You are in control; let them know it.

Use your hands to emphasize your body—run them over your breasts, trace the smooth contours of your legs, or sexily ruffle your hair.

Keep your routine lively by mixing it up as much as possible. Switch among slow moves, fast moves, pole moves, and floor moves. Always keep them guessing!

Buy a Peekaboo Dance Pole. It goes up anywhere with no screws, nuts, or bolts, and is ideal for beginners who want to pole dance in their own homes or at parties. You can slink, shimmy, and pose around it to develop all kinds of sexy moves.

Have a professional pole installed. There are numerous professional poles on the market. They're usually more expensive and require expert fitting, but they will provide you with more stability should you want to progress to full swings, climbs, and inverted moves.

Above all else, make sure you're having lots and lots of flaunty fun!

Performing a Peekaboo Pole Dance

Every Peekaboo Pole Dancing session should begin with a warm-up routine and end with a cool-down session. It's important to prepare your body and stretch those sexy muscles to minimize the chance of injury or strain.

Remember, pole dancing is not suitable for pregnant women, or for people with concerns about their health. Those who are unsure should consult a doctor.

Before you start, it's important to get into the right frame of mind. Are you feeling like Girly Girl Pink? Are you out with the girls? Are you Party Girl Purple about to get a party going full swing? Maybe you're Bad Girl Black about to get up to some mischief in the bedroom. Whoever you are, it's important that you are confident, comfortable, and ready to enjoy yourself.

Next, think about the song you are about to dance to and perhaps about some of the Peek-a-Moves you'd like to incorporate into your dance.

Choose your favorite pole-dancing tracks to begin with. As your confidence grows, you'll get more of a feel for these songs and be able to start developing a more choreographed routine. Remember, slinky R 'n' B or heaving rock tracks are best for beginners.

Take things slow to start with—don't panic or rush around the pole. Start slow, be confident and in control, and dance at your own pace.

You should aim to incorporate between five and ten moves into each dance. The trick is to link each move with the next so that the routine flows. Try to slink around and sensually dance your way from one move to another so your routine looks seamless.

Remember, there are no strict rules or choreographed dance routines. Each dance should be different depending on the music, your mood, the setting, what you're wearing, and so on. The diagram on page 21 can be used as a loose framework, but the rest is completely up to you!

Each dance will last around three minutes.

Enjoy! The best thing about Peekaboo Pole Dancing is that it is pole dancing for fun, flaunty fun! Hopefully this book has equipped you with everything you need to have just that. For more information and a whole lot more flaunty fun, you can reach us at peekaboopalace.com.

Good luck and have fun!

Peekaboo

Everyone at the Peekaboo Palace!

You've got it, so flaunt it!

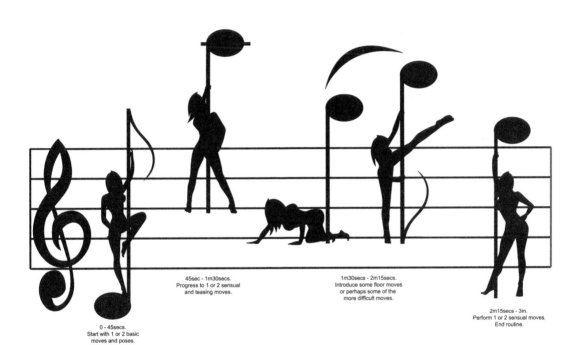

0 - 45secs.
Start with 1 or 2 basic
moves and poses.

45sec - 1m30secs.
Progress to 1 or 2 sensual
and teasing moves.

1m30secs - 2m15secs.
Introduce some floor moves
or perhaps some of the
more difficult moves.

2m15secs - 3m.
Perform 1 or 2 sensual moves.
End routine.

Getting to Know You

Start off slow and easy with this naughty little number. Performing this move will help you get to grips with the pole using a very simple, touchy-feely approach.

Put on some slow music and take the time to familiarize yourself with your tall, shiny new dance partner.

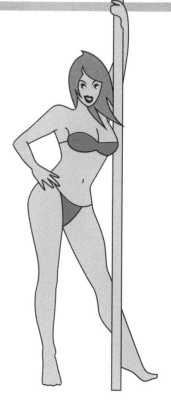

1. Don't be nervous or shy; be bold and confident as you hold your dance pole.

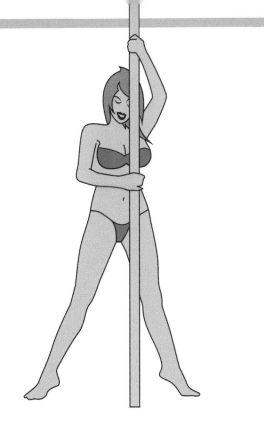

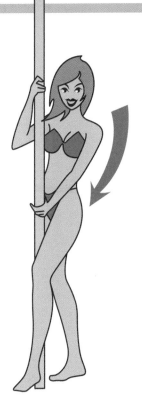

2. Dancing slowly and intimately, feel your way around it using more than just your fingers.

3. Slide your hands up and down the pole as you gently sway from side to side. Pleased and teased to meet you!

Swing It, Sister

Let's get things started nice and slow. This cheeky little move will make sure you draw all eyes to your shapely curves. It requires only a little effort, but the results will say a lot.

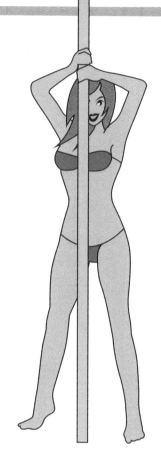

1. Start by standing seductively behind your pole, holding it with both hands.

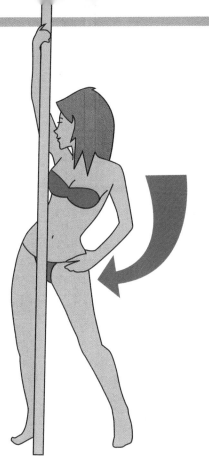

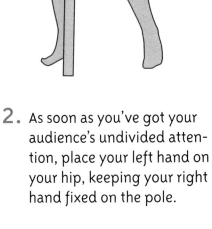

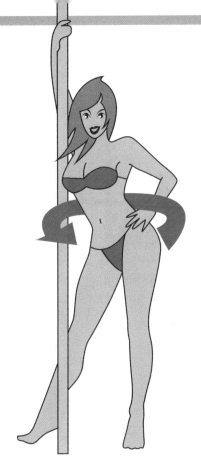

2. As soon as you've got your audience's undivided attention, place your left hand on your hip, keeping your right hand fixed on the pole.

3. Now roll your hips in a circular motion. Gently gyrate, and put a little bit of sexy swing into it!

Little Miss Wiggle

Here's a very simple move where you can really work your wiggly magic and charm your audience.

A cheeky wiggle is a great way to Miss Behave!

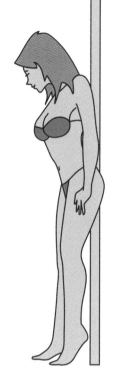

1. Start by standing with your back to the pole (not against it) with your hands by your sides.

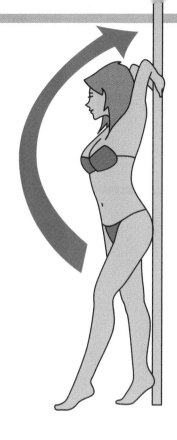

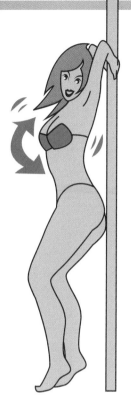

2. Now bring your hands up and lightly grasp the pole from behind.

3. Keeping your weight on your legs, slowly bend your knees, push your breasts out, and give them a little shake. Who's a little Miss Naughty?

Seamed Stocking

This inviting, intimate move will probably give you a reputation as the ultimate seductress.

Who knows? With the right amount of practice you could become the next Gypsy Rose Lee!

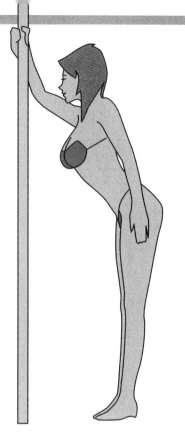

1. Start with your left hand by your side and your right holding the pole.

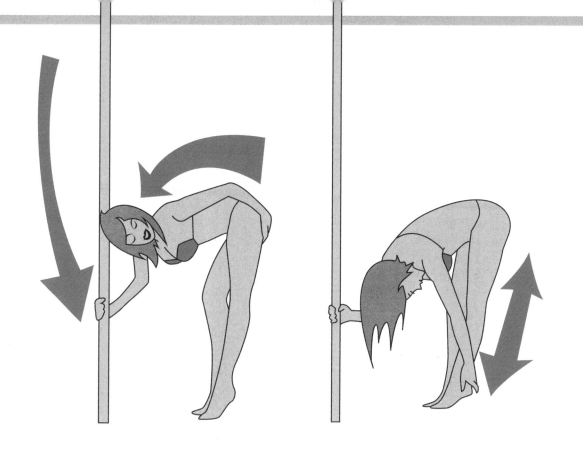

2. As you slide your right hand down the pole, gracefully bend over and hoist your sexy butt in the air.

3. Now slowly trace your fingers up and down the back of your seamed stockings. It's going to be sheer pleasure for you and your audience.

29

Kissy Kissy

This move is designed to give your audience a treat. So pucker up those luscious lips and get ready to blow kisses right, left, and center.

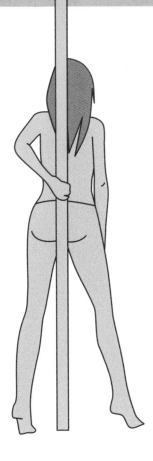

1. Stand with your back to the pole (not leaning against it).

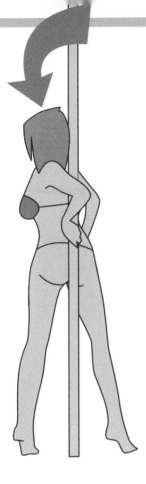

2. Place your left hand on the pole behind you.

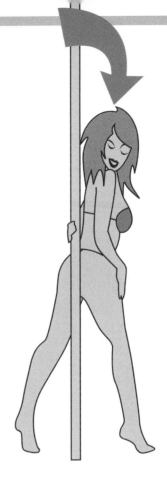

3. Keeping your legs in the same position, move your body from left to right as you turn and blow kisses over your shoulders.

Teasy Does It

Tease them and please them with this titillating little number.

Make sure you maintain eye contact all the way through. Don't forget to pose and pout!

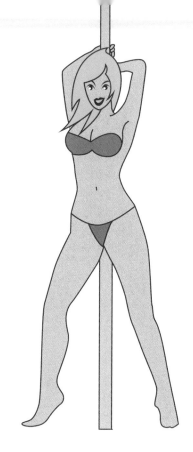

1. Start with your back to the pole, holding it behind you like you mean business.

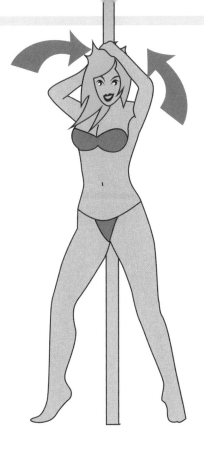

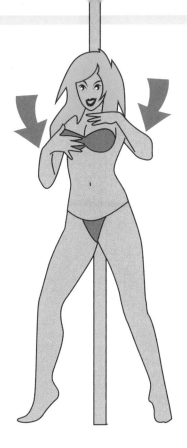

2. Now transfer your hands from the pole to your hair. Play with your hair and gently tease your luscious locks.

3. Move your hands down to your breasts and gently stroke them while rolling your hips from side to side. Getting this move right should be easy, teasy!

The Strut

This little move requires you to find your inner showgirl. You're on parade and everyone has come out to see, so give them your best strut.

Get ready to stand and deliver.

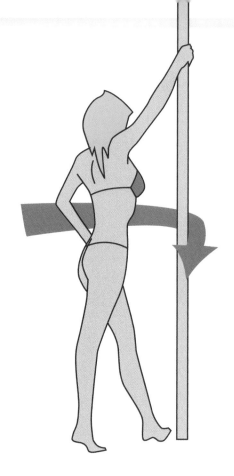

1. Start with your right hand on the pole and your left hand on your hip.

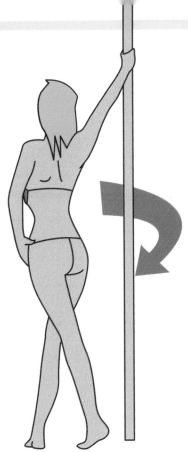

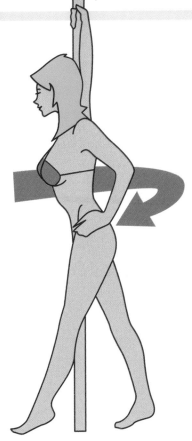

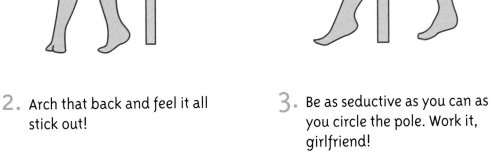

2. Arch that back and feel it all stick out!

3. Be as seductive as you can as you circle the pole. Work it, girlfriend!

Sexy Lady

To be a sexy lady you need three things—attitude, poise, and elegance. And this move certainly requires all three.

Now, don't forget your manners.

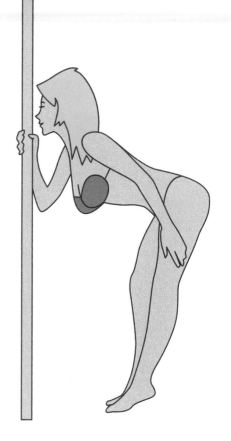

1. Start with your right hand lightly on the pole (you should not need the pole for support) and your right leg slightly bent forward.

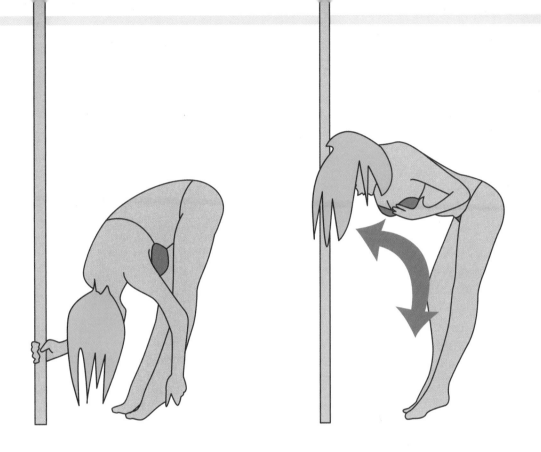

2. As you slide your hand elegantly down the pole, bend over.

3. To finish, trace your left hand seductively over your thighs, breasts, and face.

See Saw

This intimate move is perfect if you want to heat things up a little. You can make it as cheeky and fun as you like.

Rub your body up the right way.

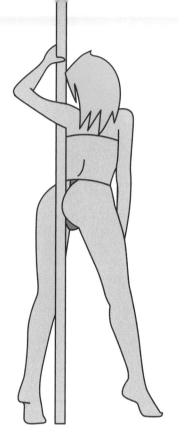

1. Start with your back to the pole (not leaning against it), with your feet positioned apart and a short distance away. Lightly grasp the pole with your left hand.

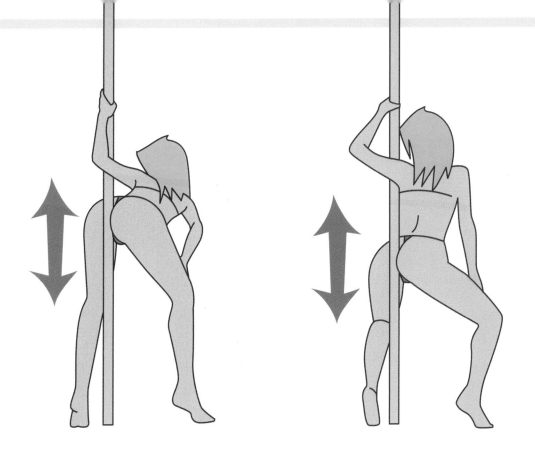

2. Keeping all your weight on your feet, bend your knees forward so that your butt is lightly touching the pole.

3. With the pole as a guide, work your butt up and down to the beat of the music. Work it, girlfriend, work it!

Get Down On It

This lively, groovy move is great for showing off your luscious legs and beautiful booty! Get the most from it by putting on some bootylicious beats.

Ramp up the music and ramp up the raunchy!

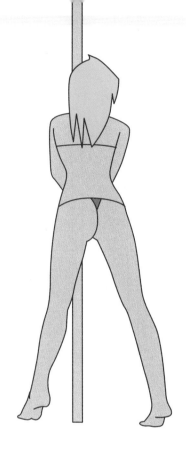

1. With your back facing the audience, hold the pole at waist height.

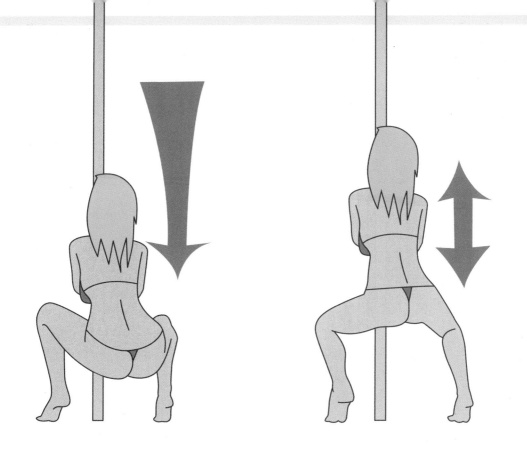

2. Making sure you keep your weight on your legs, gently lift up your butt and slowly slide seductively down the pole.

3. Move up and down the pole at a pace that suits your mood, the music, and your leg muscles!

The Head Roller

This is an easy move that's great for warming things up. It's time to have some fun and get the party started.

Let the music kick in and do your foxy thang . . .

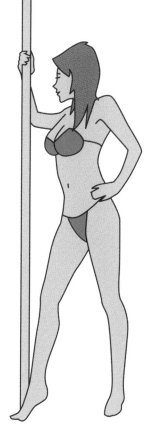

1. Start by holding the pole with your right hand.

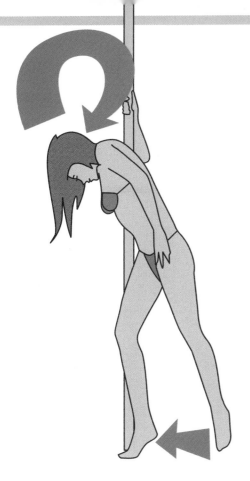

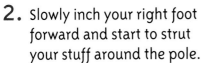

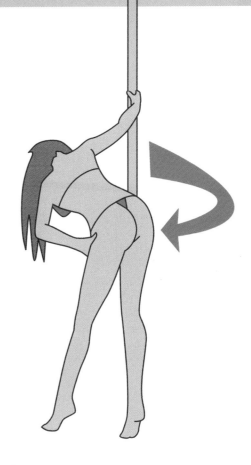

2. Slowly inch your right foot forward and start to strut your stuff around the pole.

3. Now roll your head around your shoulders and you'll soon have all heads in the room turning!

The Tail Feather

This move is great for the less agile among us. It works if you want to be a true seductress and show off your raunchy rear.

Be the hostess with the mostess!

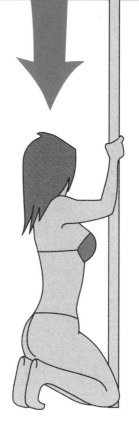

1. Start with your right hand on the pole; then slowly move down to your knees.

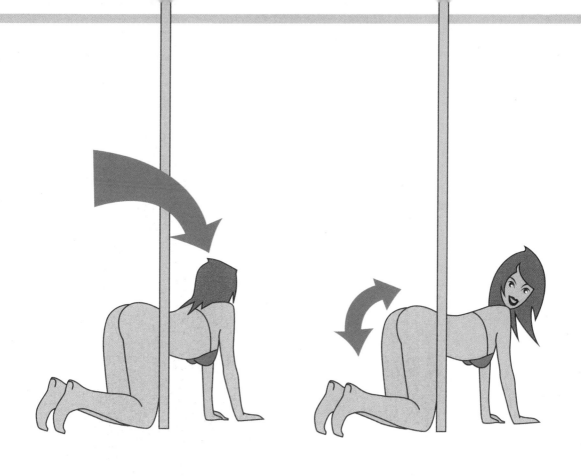

2. Now place your hands on the floor and lean your body out.

3. To finish, arch your back and jiggle your butt around.

Hip Hip Hooray!

This is a simple, fun move that's just great for showing off all your body bumps.

If you've got it, flaunt it!

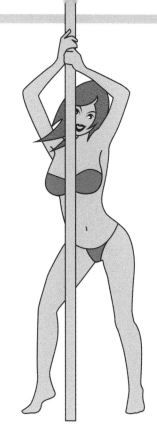

1. Stand facing your pole, holding on to it with your hands just above your head.

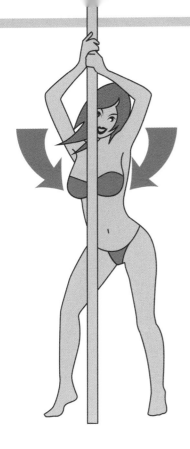

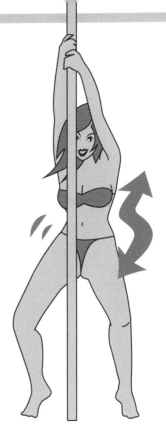

2. Now push your breasts in to the pole. Then move your hips and follow with your stomach.

3. Repeat this motion over and over to create sexy body waves. Remember, it's all in the hips.

The Party Animal

Every party girl has a party animal inside her. This move will certainly show your audience your wildest streak. Become a creature not to be messed with!

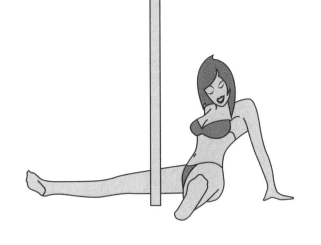

1. Start by sitting on the floor with your legs apart behind your pole. Put your arms behind you and push out your flirtatious assets.

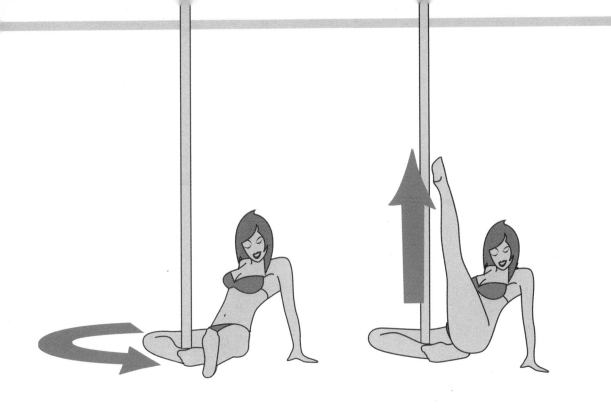

2. Curl your right leg around the pole.

3. Lift your left leg up alongside the pole (not touching it) and then stroke the inside of your left leg from your ankle right down to your inner thigh. Grrrr!

Crouching Splits

Party on down with this little party piece. It requires good coordination and strong leg muscles.

Can you be a hit with the splits?

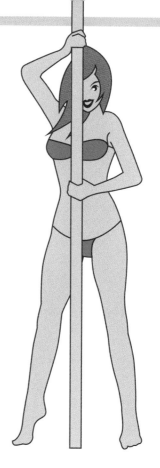

1. Start by standing behind the pole, with your feet apart, lightly grasping it with both hands.

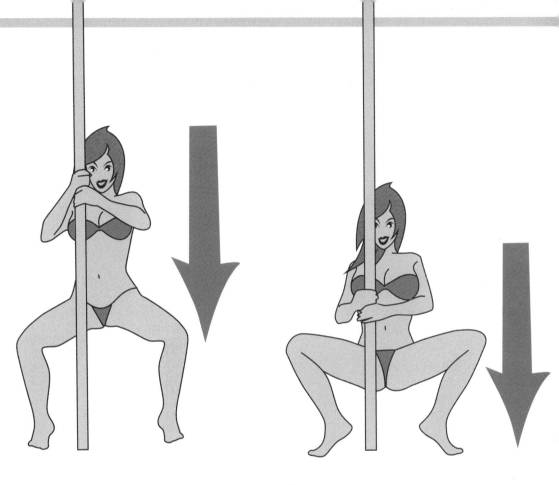

2. Bring your hands together and move slowly downward, letting your legs do the work.

3. As you get farther down, let your knees bend outward and your legs take your weight. It's time to head sexy south.

Hair Swing

Time to swing into action. This move requires you to turn up the music and let your hair down. Use a steady stance and hold on!

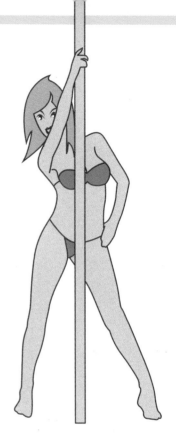

1. Stand behind your pole, but don't lean on it, with your right arm grasping it above your head.

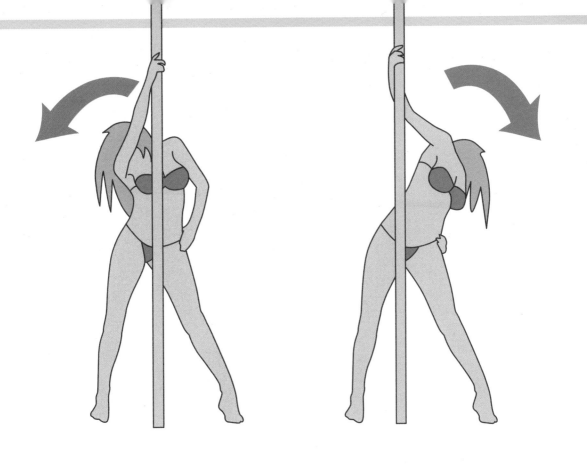

2. Place your left hand on your hip and look like you mean business.

3. Roll your head from left to right. Swing it, sister!

The Slide Show

The slower you perform this move, the sexier it is. Your hips will naturally sway as you move your knees.

Draw the curtains closed and start your slide show.

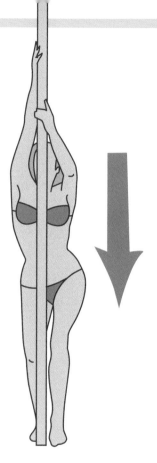

1. Start by lightly holding the pole with your right hand a little above your left.

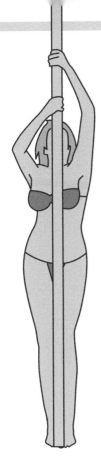

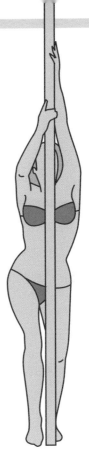

2. Now slowly slide both hands down the pole. Then slide them up and over each other to create the illusion that you're seductively sliding (or slithering) down the pole.

3. Add to the illusion by bending your knees and sashaying from side to side in a smooth, seductive manner. This is one slide show your audience won't want to miss.

Up Close and Personal

This is a provocative move that requires you step forward and get closer to your audience.

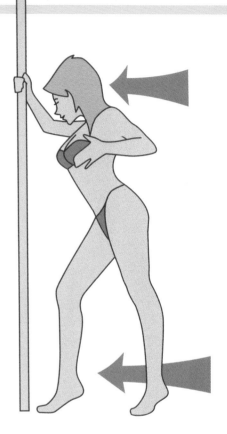

1. Stand to the side of the pole and hold it with your right hand.

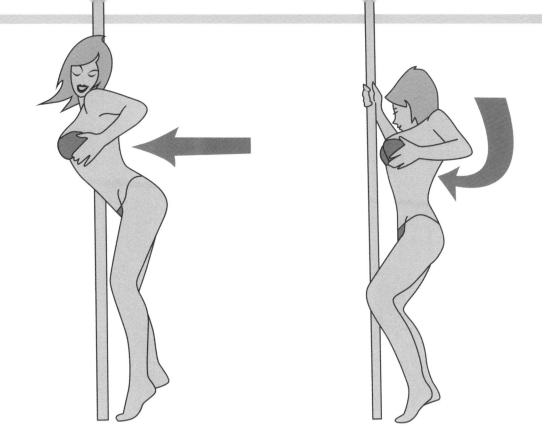

2. Gently touch your left breast with your left hand and roll your breast forward.

3. Shimmy slightly as you move toward your audience. How close is close enough? You decide.

Wiggle Wiggle

What will you shake, wiggle, or jiggle? This move encourages you to wag and wiggle your body as much as you want.

Start with a tremble and build to an earthquake.

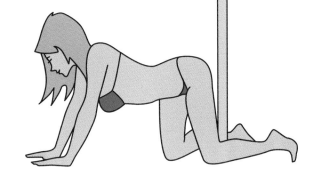

1. Start on all fours on the floor with your ankles on either side of the pole.

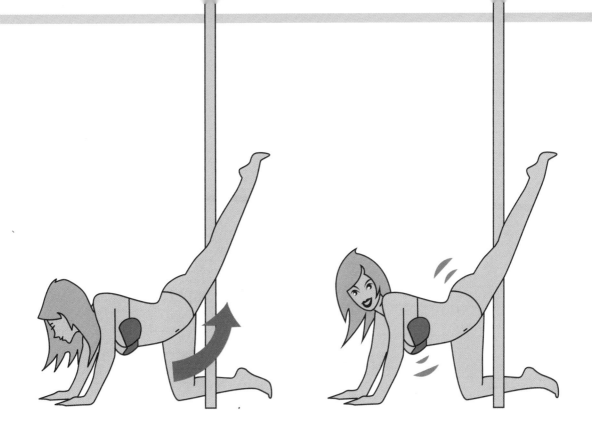

2. Hoist your left leg up.

3. Now you're in the perfect position to shake your booty or your boobs.

Boogie On Down

This move is 100 percent bootylicious.

As you boogie to the beat, remember to keep your balance and let your legs do all the work.

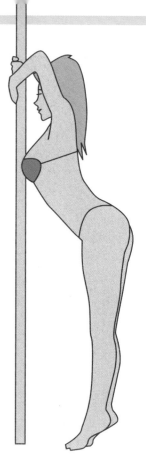

1. Start with your hands lightly grasping the pole in front of you.

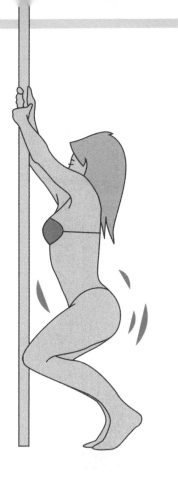

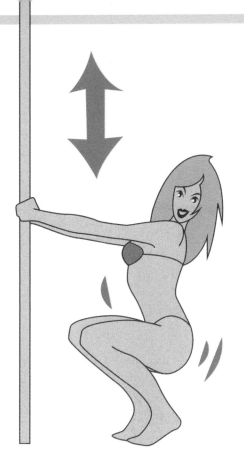

2. Keeping your balance, let your legs take your weight as you slowly move down the pole, shaking your booty from side to side.

3. Now turn to face your audience and stick your butt out. Continue to boogie all the way down and back up again. Make tonight Boogie night with a capital B.

The Tiger Crawl

This is a very sexy floor move that shows you're not scared to be a sexy beast in the bedroom.

It's time to take your audience on a wild adventure!

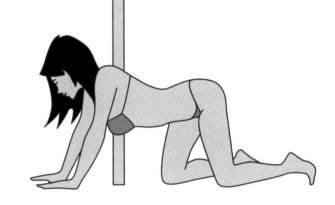

1. Start by getting down on all fours by your pole.

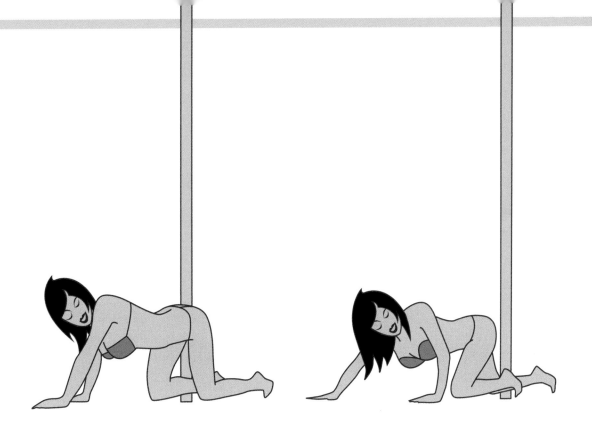

2. Move your right knee and your left arm forward. Follow with your left knee and right arm.

3. Crawl around the pole like the untamed animal you are. Easy, tiger!

Peekaboo to You

This is a cheeky little move that'll show off your legs and will inject a little fun into your routine.

It's a floor move that should be performed facing your audience.

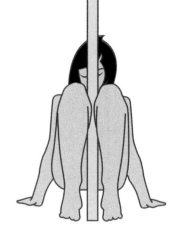

1. Start by sitting on the floor with the pole between your knees and your hands down by your sides.

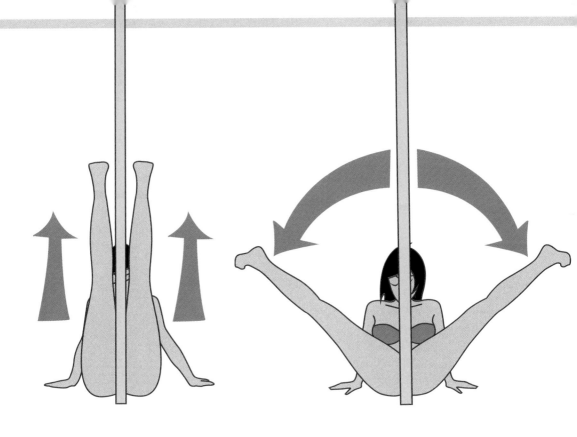

2. Now, leaning back and transferring your weight onto your hands, slowly lift your legs into a vertical position.

3. Hide behind your legs for a beat, then drop them open and peek out at your audience. Well, hello there!

Cat
Stretch

A very feline move that shows off all your curvaceous curves. Charm them by moving and crawling in slow motion—soon everyone will be falling for this pussycat.

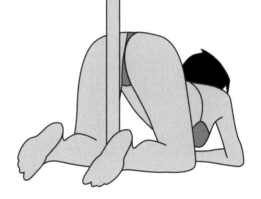

1. Start on the floor on your knees and elbows. Your butt should be gently resting against your pole (take care not to push back against the pole).

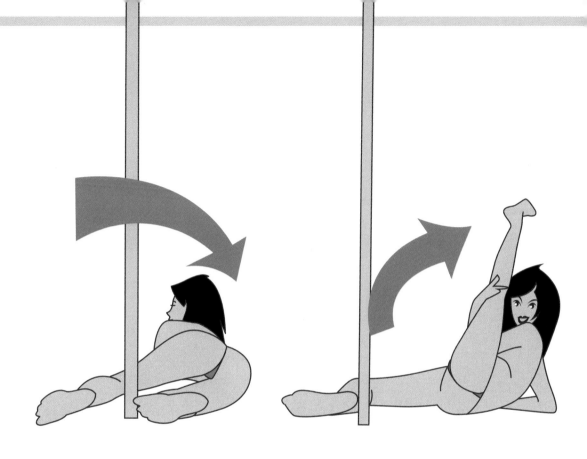

2. Transfer your weight onto your right-hand side and roll over.

3. Complete this move by lifting your left leg up to the sky. Purrr . . . fect!

Squeeze to Please

This seductive and intimate move will make the most of your breast assets. Just relax, go with the music, and simply get into the groove.

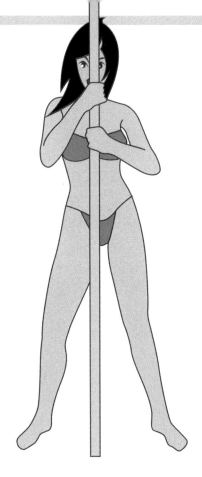

1. Start by standing behind the pole, holding on to it.

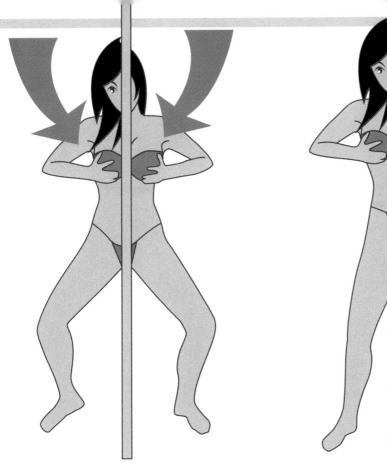

2. Next, move your hands toward your breasts and gently push them together.

3. Slide slowly up and down the pole in time with the music.

How's This for Thighs?

This intimate move is very simple and will drive your audience crazy.

The trick is to maintain eye contact with your audience at all times, then teasingly tempt them into looking at your inner thighs.

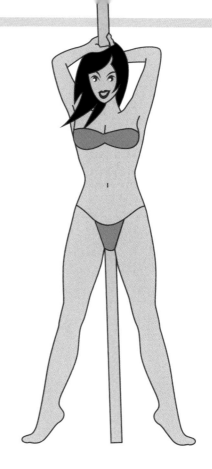

1. Start standing with your back to the pole (not leaning against it) while holding it with both hands behind your head.

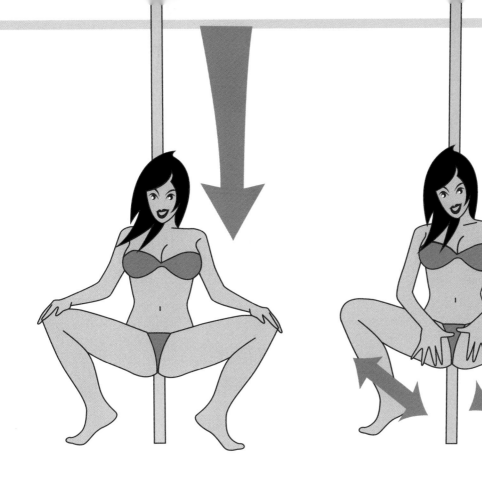

2. Now open your legs outward. Keeping your weight
   on your feet at all times,
   slowly move down the pole.
   Don't lean on the pole; let
   your legs take control.

3. Maintain eye contact at all
   times and gently caress your
   inner thighs with your fingers. Become a little Miss
   Bad Behavior.

The Acrobat

This move requires agility and balance; it resembles the type of move normally performed by trapeze artists and acrobats. Hold on tight, though; you'll be performing without a safety net!

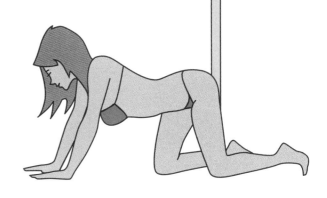

1. Start on all fours, facing away from your audience, and with the pole between your legs. All your body weight should be on your hands, knees, and legs.

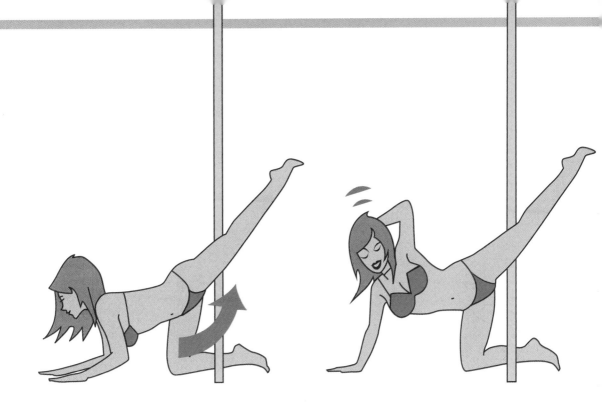

2. Transferring your weight to your right leg, slowly and seductively lift your left leg up into the air so it comes diagonally across, barely touching the pole.

3. Keeping your weight on your right side, move your left hand up to behind your head, hold still, and let them admire your newfound talent!

73

On Your Knees and Play

This knee trembler is a great way to give your legs a workout and show off all your cheeky curves.

Simply let your top half sway and play while your bottom half does all the work.

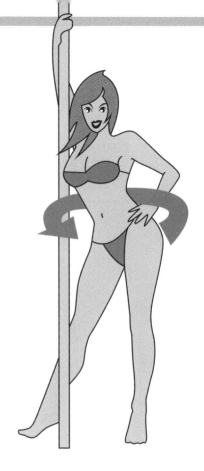

1. Start by standing behind the pole. Lightly grasp it with your right hand and put your left hand on your hip.

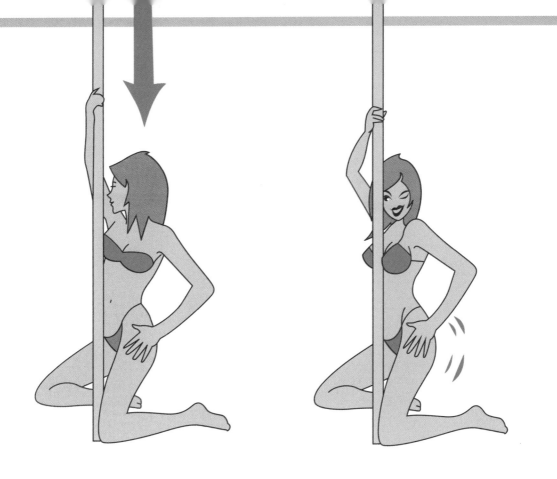

2. Slowly and seductively move down onto your knees, letting your legs take all your weight.

3. Now shake and shimmy to the music. Move your right hand up and down the pole and shake your booty. It's Peekaboo Playtime!

Easy Teasy

This move will make sure you stand out at any party. The sways will cause a sensation. Are you ready to be a total knockout?

Make it a party they'll never, ever forget!

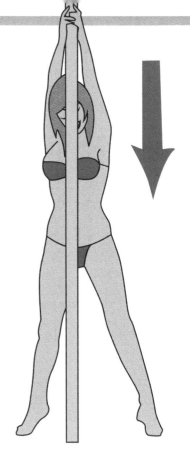

1. Start with your body stretched out, and your hands up high, lightly grasping the pole.

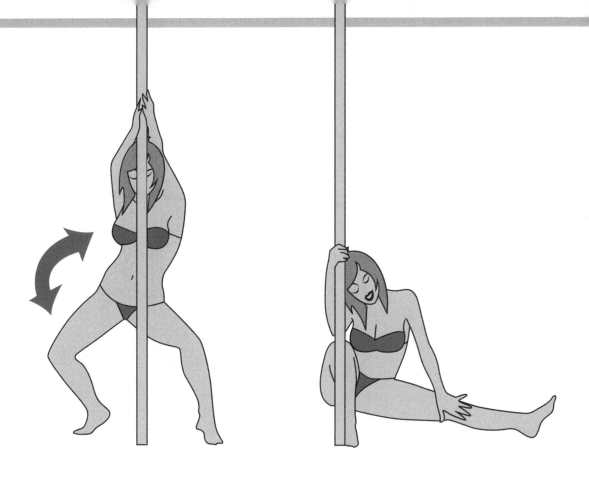

2. Now, letting your legs take your weight, slowly bend your knees outward and start to sway your hips.

3. As you sway, move down the pole and allow your right leg to take all your body weight. Finish with your butt on the floor with your left leg stretched out. It's easy, when you know how.

The Caress

This playful move teasingly guides your audience to look wherever you want them to.

Doing a little flaunty, fun fondle will drive your audience wild.

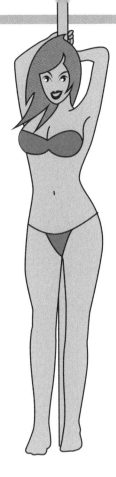

1. Start by standing with your back to the pole (not against it), with your hands lightly grasping it behind your head.

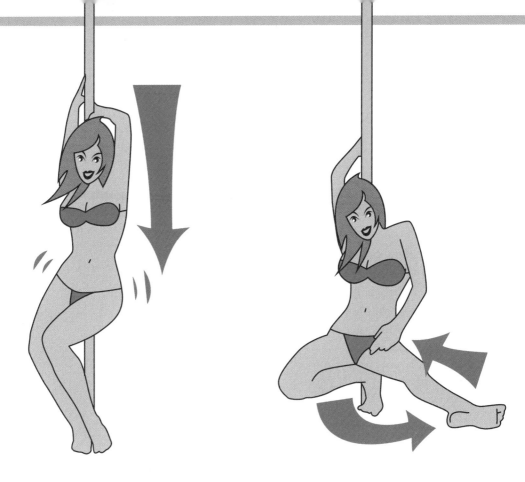

2. Slowly and seductively arch your back and roll your hips from side to side as you move down the pole. Don't lean against the pole; let your legs do all the work.

3. Transfer all your weight onto your right leg as you slowly slide your left leg out in front of you. Finish by gently caressing the contours of your body with your left hand. Smooth!

Kick Ass

Keep your audience on their toes and surprise them with this cheeky little kick. This move is great when performed repeatedly along to the beat. You can also use it as a way to punctuate the end of a seductive routine.

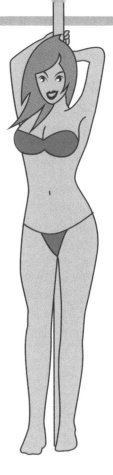

1. Stretch out those girly-girl curves and start with your back to the pole (not leaning against it) while lightly grasping it behind your head.

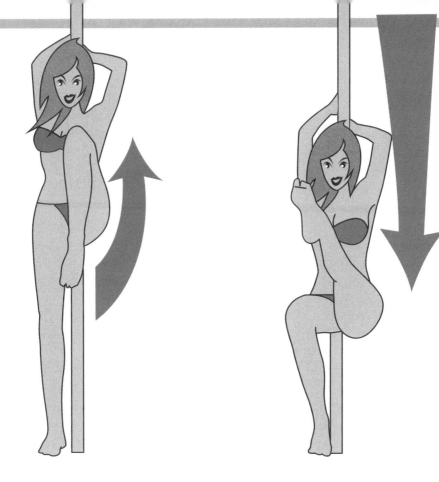

2. Transferring all your weight onto your right leg, lift your left up off the floor and pull it tight toward your chest.

3. Now do the unexpected. Kick out your left leg and slowly move down the pole to the floor. Remember, don't lean back against the pole; your right leg should do the all the work. Even a girly girl has gotta get her kicks!

Check Me Out

This is a very cheeky little number. It's very brave and bold, and will have everybody's undivided attention.

It's also your chance to show your audience that there's a little more to you than meets the eye.

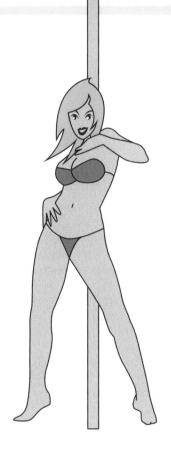

1. Start with your back to the pole and flaunt everything you've got.

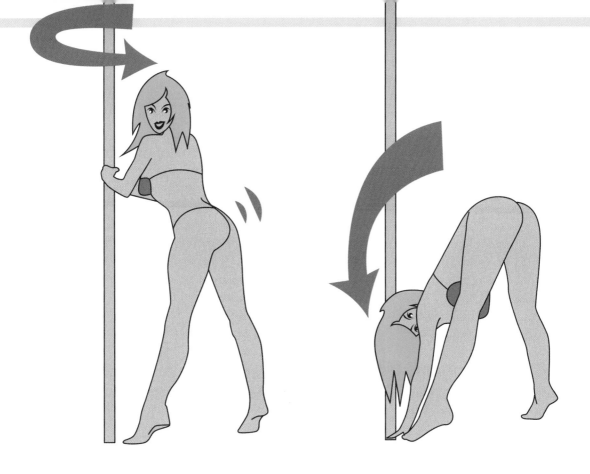

2. Now turn, hold the pole, and show that there's a lot more behind, too! Seductively roll your hips from side to side.

3. Slowly bend over and stroke the back of your leg, so they can check it all out!

Hand Spin

This move really stretches your upper body. It may seem quite complicated at first—but practice makes perfect!

Take it nice and slow and let yourself go . . .

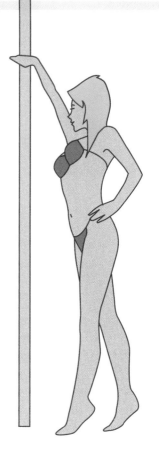

1. To start, lightly grasp the pole with your right hand, this time with your palm facing upward. Hold it between your thumb and forefinger, at all times keeping your weight on your feet.

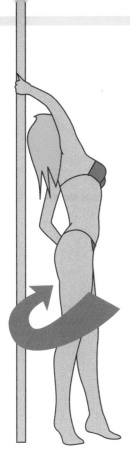

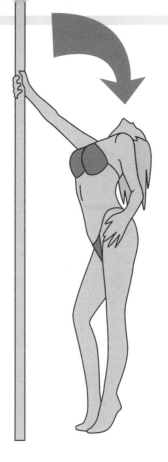

2. The next part requires a bit of skill. Turn your body around and spin under your right arm. As you do so, your hand should turn into an upright position.

3. Finish by slowly and carefully tilting your head back (keeping your balance at all times). Everyone likes a show-off!

Bend Over Backward

Not only is this floor move a bit physical; it's also very saucy, so it's up to you how far you go. It requires good balance and coordination, but if you aim to please, then bending over backward will certainly do the trick!

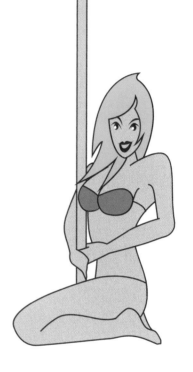

1. Start on your knees at the base of the pole. Lightly drape an arm around it and get comfortable. Your legs should be at either side of the pole, but not touching it.

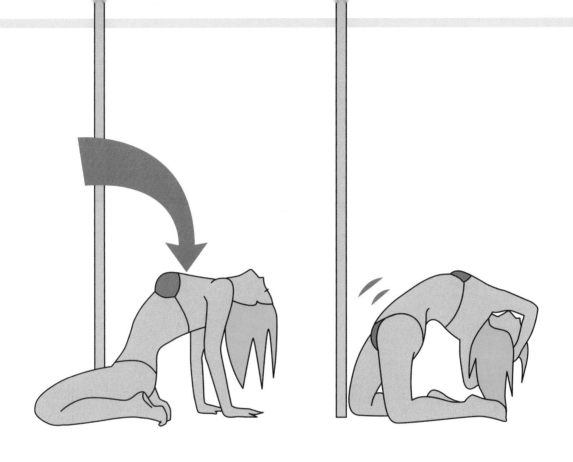

2. Let your hands take some of your body weight as you lean back and place them on the floor behind you.

3. Now push your pelvis up skyward and rock back and forth, flaunting your flexibility as you go.

The Poser

This is a great move if you love being the center of attention. Make sure you are as saucy as you can possibly be.

It's time to take center stage, strike a pose, and get the attention you so thoroughly deserve.

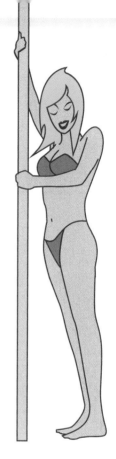

1. To start, stand a little to the left of the pole, lightly grasping it up high with your right hand and at chest height with your left.

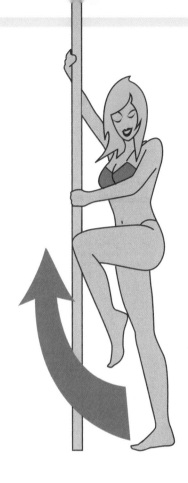

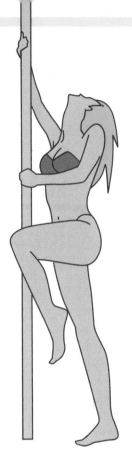

2. Transferring all your weight onto your right leg, gently lift your left knee up and hold it.

3. Now slowly and carefully tilt your head back (keeping your balance at all times) and strike a pose. Come on, vogue!

The Body Beautiful

This move is a sure way to release any inhibitions you have and to show off all your sexy curves. It's guaranteed to leave you feeling liberated, alive, and goddamn sexy.

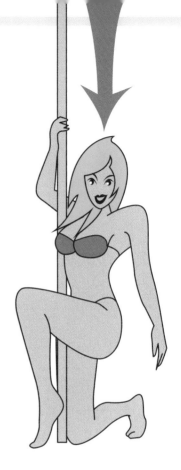

1. Start kneeling with your right hand holding the pole.

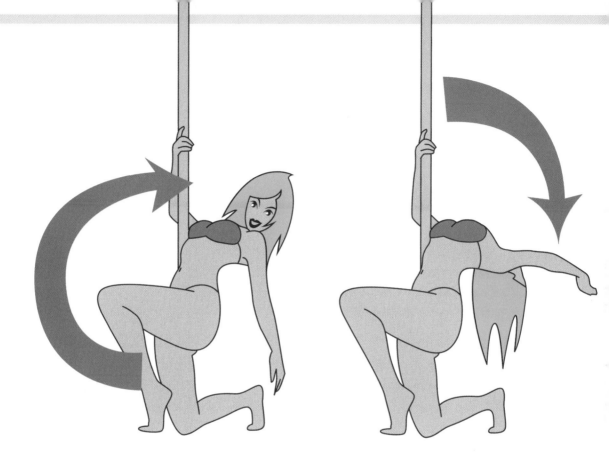

2. Slowly make your move. Come down slowly, putting your weight onto your right bended knee.

3. Finish by slowly and carefully tilting your head and left arm back and out (remember to keep your weight on your legs and your balance at all times). Don't it feel good?

The Wink and Smile

This is a more advanced party trick and should be performed only when you are confident you have developed good balance and pole-dancing posture.

It's an ideal way to get noticed at a party and will definitely leave a lasting impression.

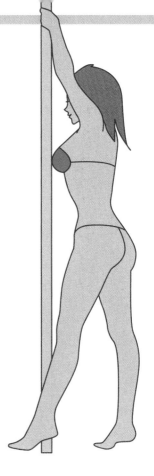

1. Start standing beside the pole, lightly grasping it with your left hand.

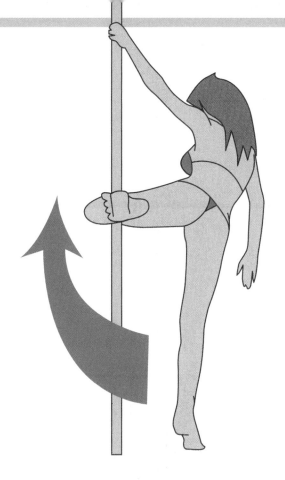

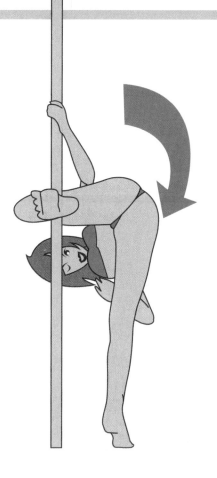

2. Transferring all your weight onto your right leg, gently wrap your left leg around the pole and slowly lean over. Make sure you keep your balance at all times and your weight on your right foot.

3. Now simply look back at your audience and give them your wickedest wink and sexiest smile!

The High Flyer

This move is quite advanced but will show your audience you're one clever cookie. It's a smart move that's great for showing off your legs.

If you possess a lot of ambition—get to it!

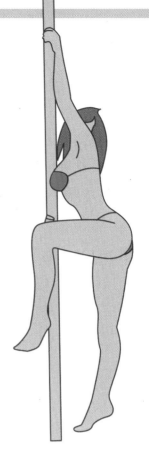

1. Start by giving your audience a profile. Lightly grasp the pole with your left hand and raise your left leg up alongside it.

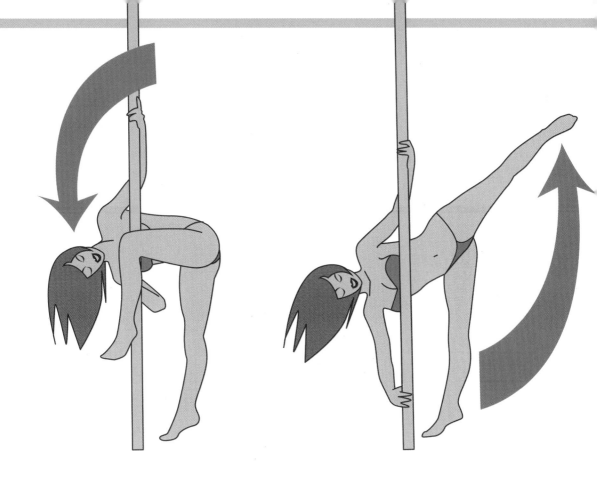

2. Next, lean to your right side. Keeping all your body weight on your right foot, lean across and to the right of the pole. Be sure not to lean over too far!

3. Without using the pole for balance, just lightly grasp the pole, stand on your right foot, and lift your left leg out. Now, that is what's called a good presentation!

The Kinky Kick

This isn't just any ordinary kicking move; this is a Kinky Kick with a capital K.

Performing this move is a great way to show off your legs and butt.

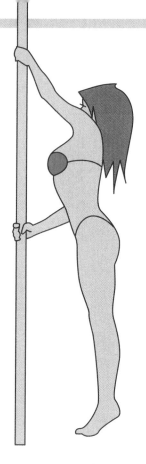

1. Start by lightly grasping the pole with your left hand up high and your right hand at waist level.

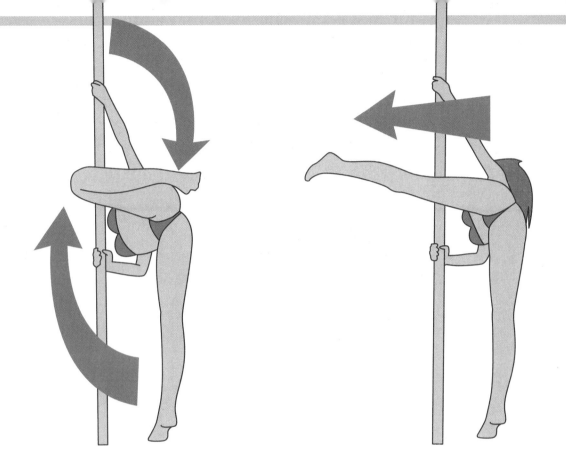

2. Transferring all your weight onto your right leg, slowly lean over to the right as you bring your left leg up. Make sure you keep your balance at all times, but take care not to use the pole to aid your balance.

3. Holding this position, slowly and seductively stretch your left leg right out. Work all those kinky kinks out of your sexy system.

The Seductress

This is an especially seductive move with a bit of a sexy kick at the end.

It requires you to maintain eye contact with your audience, and then take it by sexy surprise.

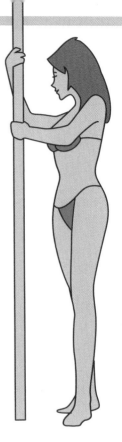

1. Seduce your audience with some light slinking and swaying around the pole.

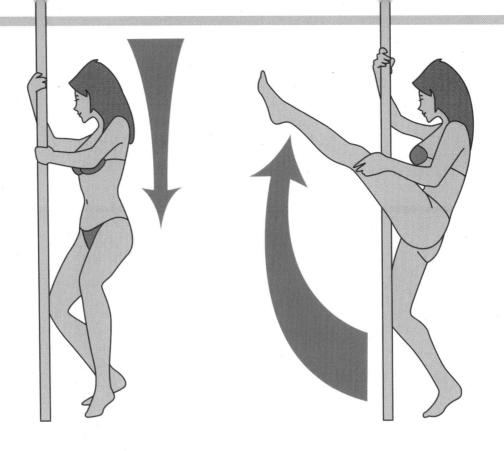

2. Looking passionately into their eyes, continue to slink a little lower by bending your knees and letting your legs take your weight.

3. Maintaining eye contact at all times, go in for the kill by swooping your left leg up for a grand finale. Remember, don't lean back against the pole; keep your balance and let your right leg do the all the work.

The Can-Can

This advanced little number is the ultimate move to make at a party. It takes real skill, as you have to be quite flexible and steady to pull it off.

Can-Can you do it?

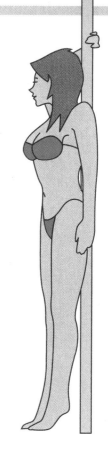

1. Start with your back to the pole (not leaning against it), with your right hand lightly grasping it behind your head.

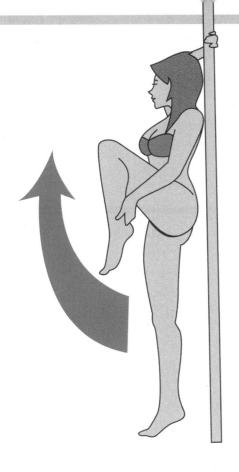

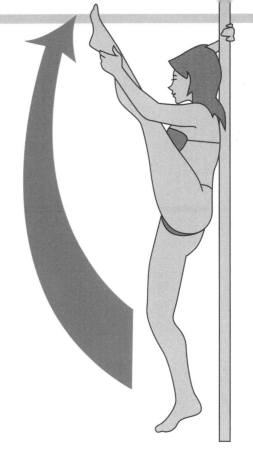

2. Transfer all your weight to your right foot and lift up your left knee. Remember, keep your balance and don't lean back against the pole; your right leg should take all your weight.

3. Now, surprise your audience by kicking outward and holding on to your raised ankle. Can it be done? You show, girl!

The Elvis Pelvis

This is a great pelvic floor exercise for you to rock and roll to. It works the pelvis and the inner thigh.

Long live the Elvis Pelvis!

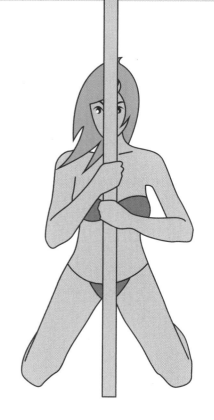

1. Start on your knees, lightly grasping the pole with both hands. Your legs should be slightly apart, one on either side of the pole.

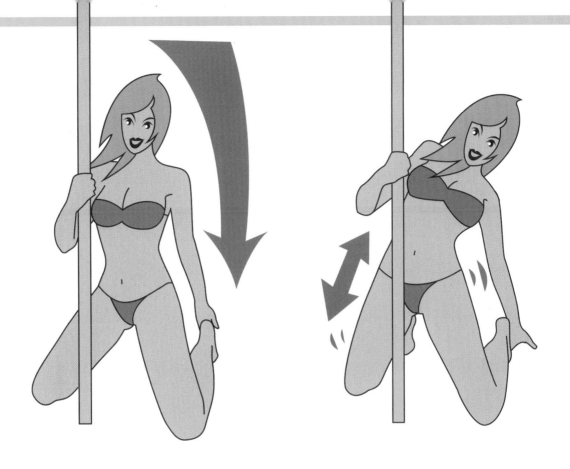

2. Slowly reach back and place your left hand on the floor behind you.

3. Letting your supporting hand and legs take all your weight, thrust your pelvis forward and shake it up and down to the beat of the music. It's time to get all shook up!

Shake, Rattle, and Roll

This move requires strong neck muscles and a good sense of balance.

It's best performed to music that has a strong beat.

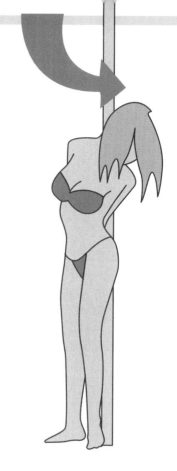

1. Start with your back to the pole, gently holding on to it from behind.

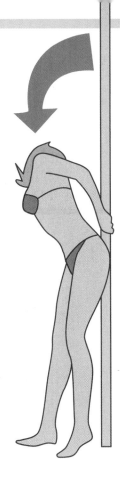

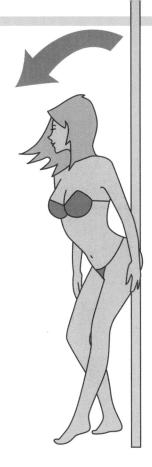

2. Begin gently swaying your head from left to right along to the music. As the music builds, you can move your head to perform sexy circles or flaunty figure eights.

3. As you get deeper and deeper into the music, let it all go, and simply shake, rattle, and roll your head along with the beat.

The Floor Slide

For this move you need good poise and balance when you go down to the floor. But remember—as you go down, your sexy reputation goes up!

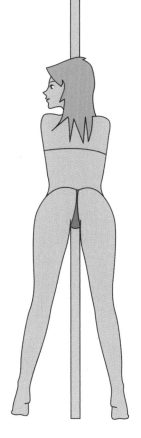

1. Start with your back and butt facing the audience.

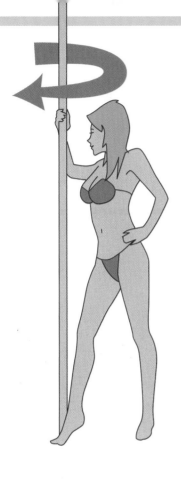

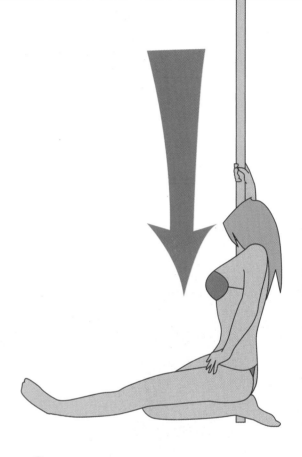

2. With your legs on either side of the pole, walk around it, holding on with your right hand.

3. Extend your left leg. With your weight on your right foot, bend your knee and glide to the floor—take care not to hang from the pole. Pull it off in one seamless move, and you'll have the whole crowd on its feet.

High Five

Gimme five! This outrageous move is sure to hit the spot.

It's one of the more advanced moves and should be performed only when you have developed good balance and pole posture.

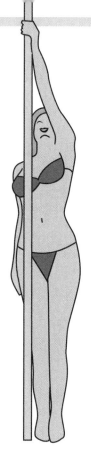

1. Start by standing behind the pole, lightly grasping it with your left hand up high.

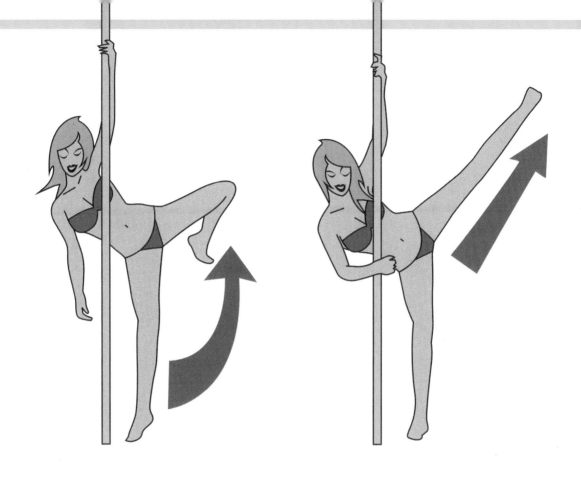

2. Carefully keeping your balance, gently lean out to the right of the pole and bring your left leg up. Be sure to keep all your weight on your standing leg at all times.

3. Slowly straighten your left leg and point it skyward. How's that for a high five!

Booty Booty

This energetic move will give your booty all the attention it craves. Get your bodacious butt out there and have some bootylicious fun!

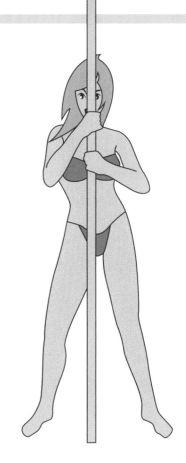

1. Start behind the pole and stick your butt out.

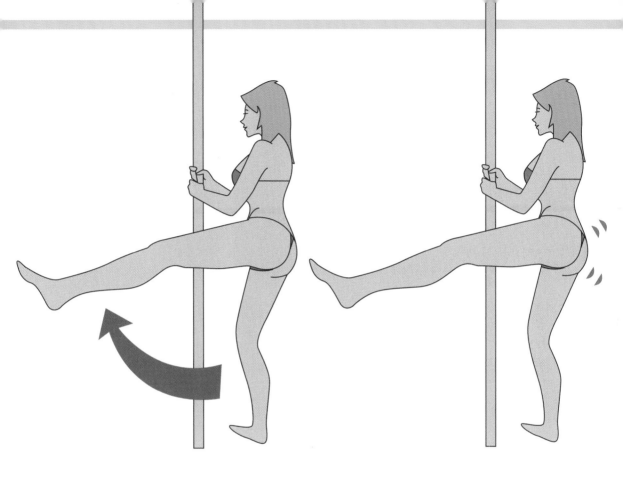

2. Lift your left leg out to the side of the pole so your butt faces your audience.

3. Now shake that booty! Absolutely bootiful!

Peep Show

This is a move for the brave and the bold . . . and for the very flexible, too. Keep it slow and keep it sexy.

It gives your audience more than just a peep; it gives them the best seat in the house!

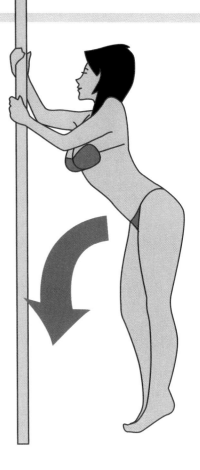

1. Start by holding the pole with both hands. Then arch your back and push out your butt.

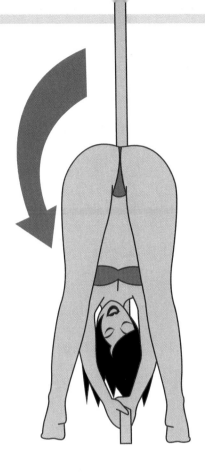

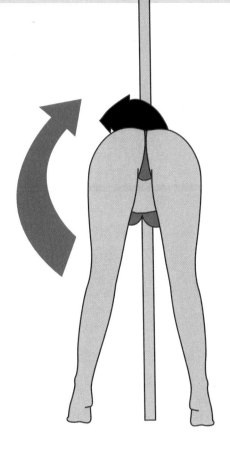

2. Now slowly slide your hands down the pole.

3. Next, slowly edge your hands back up the pole and straighten back up. If you keep it cool, you'll heat up the room.

The Wild Side

This move is not for the timid. Once you've got yourself in full swing, it's time to really turn it up and show how wild you can be.

Will you have to be tamed?

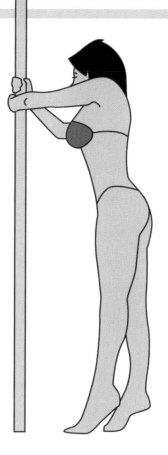

1. Stand to the side of the pole and hold it at shoulder height.

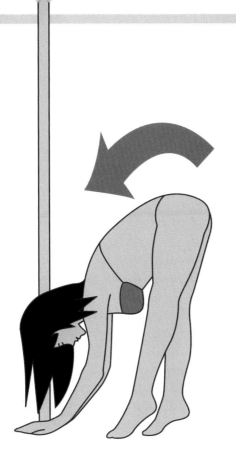

2. Release your left arm and swing down to the floor.

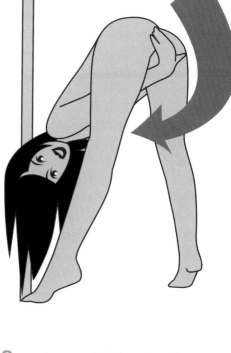

3. Take your left hand and seductively trace it from your butt to your stomach.

The Showgirl

This move is all about showing off your body. Best performed slowly and seductively to a slow or sensual song, it will stretch you to your sexy limit. How far will you go?

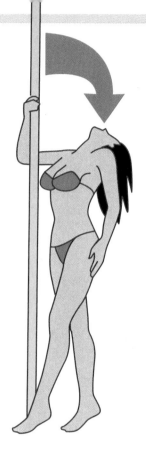

1. Start standing next to the pole, lightly grasping it with your right hand. Slowly and seductively tilt your head back and expose your neck.

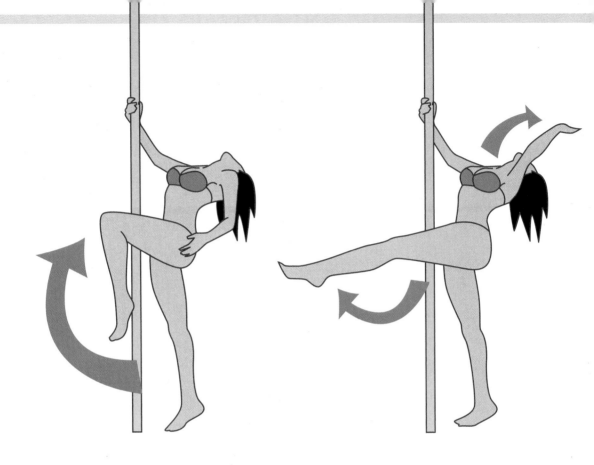

2. Keeping your balance at all times, slowly and gently lift your left leg up and out.

3. Finish by extending your leg and left arm while keeping your weight on your right foot. Keep your balance and flaunt everything you got. You show, girl!!

No Ifs
Just Butts

This intermediate move requires good poise and balance, and will definitely put your butt center stage! It works especially well when dancing to music with strong booty-shaking beats.

This move says, "Kiss my attitude!"

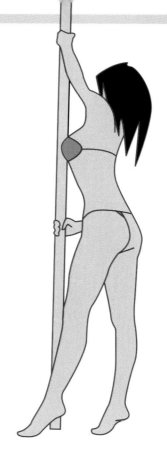

1. Start by facing the pole, lightly grasping it with your left hand at shoulder height and with your right hand at hip height.

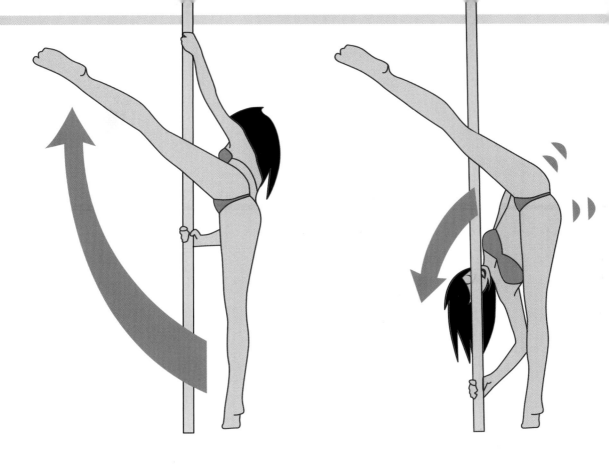

2. Transferring all your weight onto your right leg, slowly lean your body out and to the right. Lift your left leg up as high as it will go. Make sure you keep your balance at all times.

3. Now, leading with your right hand, move down the pole farther so that your butt is facing your audience. Keeping your balance and placing all your weight on your standing leg, shake and wiggle that booty!

119

Drop
Splits

This is an advanced move that should be performed only if you are already able to perform the splits. Anyone who is unsure should first practice this move as a floor move without the use of a dance pole.

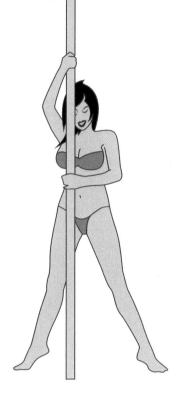

1. Stand facing your audience, lightly grasping the pole with both of your hands.

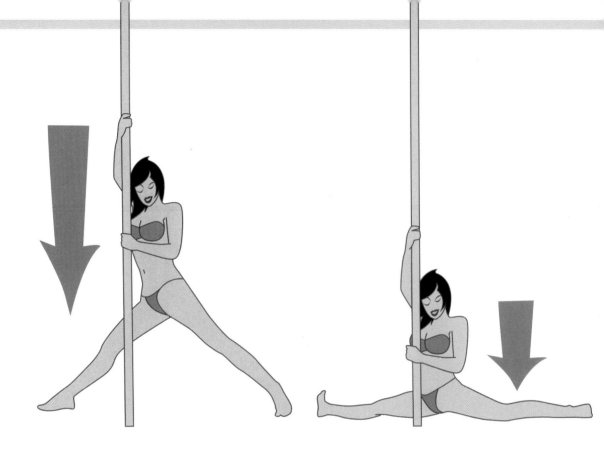

2. Keeping your torso upright at all times, start slowly lowering yourself downward into the splits position.

3. As you gently reach the bottom, take the opportunity to show off big-time!

Index